Knee Rehabilitation

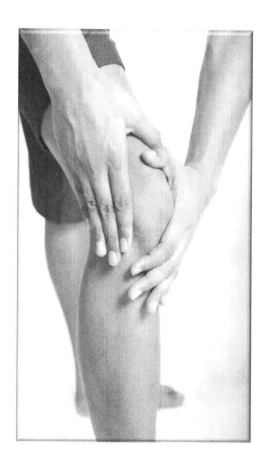

Ben Gamon
Certified Personal Trainer

ACKNOWLEDGMENTS

I'm currently working for Crunch Fitness in Los Angeles, which is the best place in the world.

I hold numerous national certifications such as:

- NASM CPT: Certified Personal Trainer through the National Academy of Sports and Medicine.
- NASM PES: Performance Enhancement Specialist.
- NASM CES: Corrective Exercise Specialist.
- NASM OPT for Prenatal.
- NASM Business Management for Fitness Professionals.
- NASM Weight Loss Management.

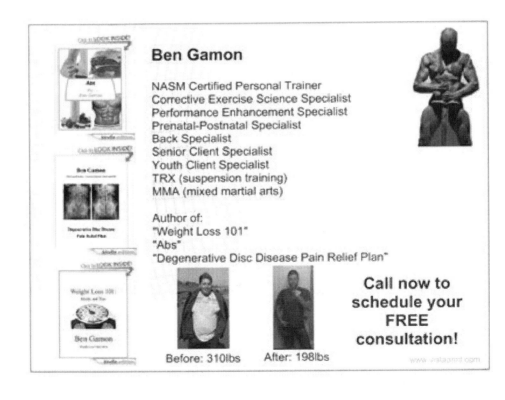

From the same Author:

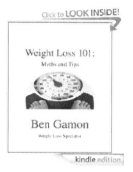
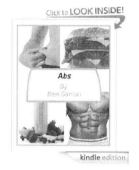
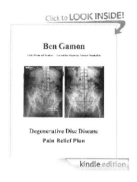
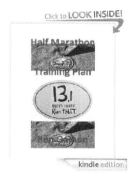
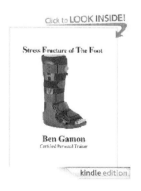

I dedicate this book to my brother Shawn.

NOTICE

This book is intended as a reference volume only, not as a medical manual. The information given here is designed to help you make informed decisions. It is not intended as a substitute for any treatment that may have been prescribed by a doctor. If you suspect that you may have a medical problem, we urge you to seek medical help. Mentions of specific companies or products in this book do not imply endorsement by the author or publisher, nor does mention of specific companies, organizations, or authorities imply that they endorse this book, its author, or its publisher.

Regardless of your condition, discuss exercise options with a doctor before beginning any new exercise program.

As with any change in lifestyle, your body will need time to adapt to your new program. During the first few weeks, you may notice changes in the way your muscles feel, your sleep patterns, or energy levels. These changes are to be expected with increased activity. However, improper exercise levels or programs may be harmful, making symptoms worse. Regardless of the exercise program you select, it's important to begin slowly and choose a program you enjoy so that you maintain it. Make exercise part of your daily routine so that it becomes a lifetime habit.

INDEX:

INTRODUCTION

CHAPTER 1: BALANCE EXERCISES

CHAPTER 2: STRETCHES

CHAPTER 3: STRENGTHENING EXERCISES

CHAPTER 4: HOME TREATMENT

CHAPTER 5: TRX FOR KNEE REHABILITATION

CONCLUSION

INTRODUCTION

Marc had injured his knee on a hiking trip in Yosemite. After consulting his family doctor, he was advised to work out on an exercise bike. This just made the knee worse, so he consulted a second doctor who sent him for physical therapy. The physical therapist referred him to a gym, where a not-so-good personal trainer put him through a rigorous program of exercise with a rowing machine, treadmill and cross-trainer. Imagine his misery when instead of his knee getting better, it swelled up. It became much more painful, and he found himself wondering if he should buy a walking cane and move to a downstairs apartment. What was going on? Marc's knee itself was making clear that the exercise regimen was inappropriate.

You see, the body follows a natural progression of healing. Each step of the rehabilitation program needs to be in sympathy with this healing process. If not, one can do a lot of harm.

Marc's trainer had him do lunges the entire time. This whole exercise regimen contributed even more to Marc's knee feeling swollen, hot, red and painful. This is called inflammation. If the knee keeps getting stressed too much, and there is no clear rehabilitation path, then the knee just gets more painful.
You need to know the dos and don'ts of exercise regimen and so should your trainer. Most of the time knee pain occurs in overweight people, but not only. Losing the extra weight should result in less pressure on the knee, which means less pain. Yes, but that's not that simple unfortunately. The swelling and the pain that occur in the knee happen to people that are not overweight as well for many different reasons; their quadriceps are underactive and need to be strengthen. Their hamstrings and calves are overactive and need to be gently stretched. Simple balance exercises as well will improve proprioception in the knee. Finally, rest, ice, compression and elevation are needed after each session to try and minimize swelling. While the inflammation settles, you may have to limit some activities and then build these activities up again gradually during the later healing stage.

Keep in mind when starting strength training that muscles act in complementary sets. For example, you need to exercise the muscles that bend the knee as well as those that straighten it. Too much emphasis on one set of muscles may lead to muscular imbalance. The quality and timing of the muscle contraction is also important in re-building muscle strength efficiently. (That's why I always focus on form and tempo over load).
Under ideal conditions, rehabilitation would progress smoothly from balance, flexibility and strength training to endurance training and then back to full activities. Moving to endurance training too early can trigger an inflammatory response with more swelling, pain, muscle inhibition and loss of the range of motion you may already have regained. This is what happened in Marc's case. He had already lost time off work, and had now wasted all his efforts in going to the gym. His knee hurt when he was driving, his knee hurt when he was standing, his knee hurt all the time.

For Marc, pushing through the pain was not going to fix his knee. It would only make things worse. With knees, repeating cycles of healing and then renewed inflammation signify that you are pushing too hard and are not being careful enough in your rehabilitation program. Back off right down again to the first stage of rehabilitation. Return your focus to dealing with the inflammation, not the strengthening or endurance. While that might seem like a step backward, it is really a step forward towards your ultimate goal of getting better. I was afraid Marc would find my rehabilitation program boring or pointless, but the truth is that after a few weeks of balance, flexing and gentle strength training he felt less to no pain in his knee; after a couple months, we moved to endurance exercises and strengthening exercises with added weights; Now, Marc's new hobby is to run marathons. My knee rehabilitation program has helped Marc improve joint mobility, muscle strength, and overall physical conditioning. Most importantly it has helped him to keep an healthy weight.

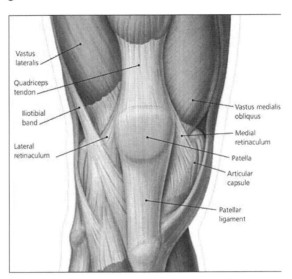

Anatomy of the knee

Exercises to avoid with knee pain:
- Running and jogging. The difference between how much force goes through your joints jogging or running, as opposed to with walking, is sometimes more than tenfold your whole body weight,
- Jump rope.
- High-impact aerobics.

Any activities with both feet off the ground at once, however briefly.

Fortunately, that leaves a lot of activities that are OK for people with knee pain and that can help keep you mobile.

Cardiovascular exercises

Good cardiovascular exercises for people with knee pain include the elliptical machine, walking, swimming, and cycling. If you can take a brisk walk, it can keep you mobile and help to reduce pain. If walking for exercise is too painful, try a recumbent bicycle. Recumbent bicycles extend the angle of the joint so that the knee and hip aren't flexing so much with each rotation, so that it might cause less strain and pain.

The foundation of endurance training is aerobic exercise, which includes any activity that increases the heart rate for a prolonged period of time. Aerobic activity conditions the heart and lungs to:

- Use oxygen to more efficiently supply the entire body with larger amounts of oxygen-rich blood
- Build stronger muscles for endurance activity

When paired with a healthy diet, aerobic activity also is fundamental for controlling weight (which is important for people with knee pain since it reduces excess pressure on affected joints) and for improving overall general health.

At first, my clients with knee pain engage in about 5 to 10 minutes of aerobic activity at least three times a week when they warm up before our training sessions. As their pain and discomfort goes away, and as we progress in our rehabilitation program, they gradually build up to 30 minutes daily. Remember to always warm up and cool down before you engage in cardiovascular activity;

Aerobic exercise should be performed at a comfortable and steady pace that allows you to talk normally and easily during the activity.

Muscle strengthening activities

By strengthening the muscles around the joints, strength training helps to take some of the load off the joints and relieves pain. The job of connective tissue is to hold things together, so losing stability in the joint is part of what's causing the pain. When you strengthen the muscles surrounding and supporting the joint, you can relieve some of the symptoms of knee pain.

Strong muscles help keep weak joints stable and comfortable and protect them against further damage. A program of strengthening exercises that target specific muscle groups can be helpful.

There are several types of strengthening exercises that, when performed properly, can maintain or increase muscle tissue to support your muscles without aggravating your joints.

Flexibility and range of motion exercises

There are a number of specific exercises that you can do to increase your flexibility and range of motion around your knees.

My clients and I focus on activities without force that bring knees through the full range of motion in a general, unforced manner, allowing the joint to lubricate itself and help to heal the pain and the swelling.

Flexibility exercises help maintain normal joint function by increasing and preserving joint mobility and flexibility. In this group of exercises, gently straightening and bending the joints in a controlled manner as far as they comfortably will go can help condition the affected joints. During the course of a flexibility exercise program, the joints are stretched progressively farther until normal or near-normal range is achieved and maintained. This helps to maintain comfort while function is preserved.

In addition to preserving joint function, flexibility exercises are an important form of warm-up and stretching, and should be done prior to performing strengthening or endurance exercises, or engaging in any other physical activity.

What are the benefits of my knee rehabilitation program?

My program will relieve the pain, discomfort and swelling around you knee. Also it will do the following:

- Help maintain normal joint movement
- Increase muscle flexibility and strength
- Help maintain weight to reduce pressure on joints
- Help keep bone and cartilage tissue strong and healthy
- Improve fitness

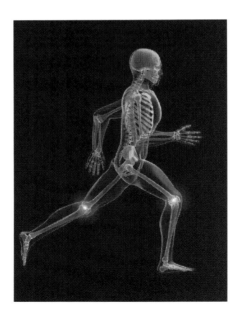

CHAPTER 1: BALANCE EXERCISES

The following balance exercises are designed to improve your balance and proprioception (joint position awareness). This is important to improve your ability to regulate shifts in your body's center of gravity while maintaining control. Balance exercises have been shown scientifically to prevent injury and are an important component of rehabilitation.

Usually, balance exercises should be performed for 5 minutes per day initially and progressed to 10-15 minutes or longer provided they do not cause or increase symptoms. Generally, you should select a range of exercises that challenge your balance without causing an increase in symptoms. A few good balance exercises are demonstrated below.

Single Leg Balance

Standing on one leg, maintain your balance . Try to hold for 1 minute. Once this exercise is too easy progress to eyes closed.

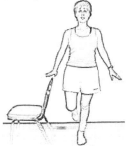

Single Leg Balance

Step up to balance

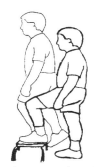

You will not be climbing the stairs. Instead, you need to place one foot on the stair or box structure, allowing the remaining free foot to dangle off to your side, above the ground next to the step.

Bend your knee, as if to step backward off of the step, but do not touch the other foot to the floor. Lower that foot as if you were going to step down on it, but then hover the foot slightly above the floor for a second before using the other leg to push back up in a standing position on the stair. If the knee supporting your weight is being challenged too much by this exercise, choose a stair or box height that is lower,

Squats on the BOSU ball

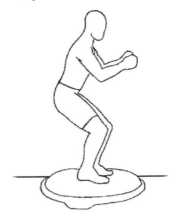

You should always start by standing on the round side of the BOSU. Stand shoulder width apart. Keep your core drawn in. You are only ready to begin when you can balance on the BOSU. You can extend your arms in front of you or to the side for balance if you want. Slowly squat down. Squat as low as you can without hurting your knees. Slowly squat back up to the balanced position and repeat.

For balance exercises, we will always progress from two feet to one foot, and from stable environment to unstable.

CHAPTER 2: STRETCHES

The following knee stretches are designed to restore movement to the knee and improve flexibility of muscles crossing the kne

Knee Bend to Straighten

Bend and straighten your knee as far as possible and comfortable pain free. Repeat 10 - 20 times.

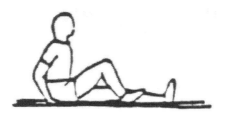

Knee Bend to Straighten

Quadriceps Stretch

(Main muscles Involved: Quadriceps - Rectus Femoris, Vastus Intermedius, Vastus Lateralis, Vastus Medialis)

The following quad stretches are designed to improve the flexibility of the quadriceps muscle. To begin with, the following quad stretches should be held for 20 seconds and repeated 4 times at a mild to moderate stretch pain free. As your flexibility improves, the exercises can be progressed by increasing the frequency, duration and intensity of the stretches, provided they are pain free.

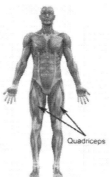

The Quadriceps Muscles

Use a chair or table for balance. Take your heel towards your bottom, keeping your knees together and your back straight until you feel a stretch in the front of your thigh. Hold for 20 seconds and repeat 4 times at a mild to moderate stretch pain-free.

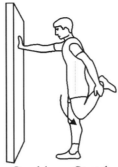
Quadriceps Stretch

Quadriceps Self Massage Exercises

The following quadriceps self-massage exercises are designed to improve the flexibility of the quadriceps and are an excellent addition to the above stretches.

Foam Roller Quadriceps Release

Place the foam roller under your quadriceps (front of your thighs) as demonstrated. Using your arms, slowly move your body forward and backwards allowing the foam roller to massage the front of your thighs. Breathe normally keeping your legs relaxed. Repeat this process for 15 – 90 seconds provided it is comfortable and does not cause pain. This exercise can be progressed by crossing your legs and massaging one thigh at a time.

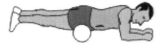
Foam Roller Quadriceps Release

Hamstring Stretch

(Main muscles involved: Hamstrings - Biceps Femoris, Semitendinosus, Semimembranosus)

The following hamstring stretches are designed to improve the flexibility of the hamstring muscles.

To begin with, the hamstring stretches should be held for 20 seconds and repeated 4 times at a mild to moderate stretch pain free. As your flexibility improves, the exercises can be progressed by increasing the frequency, duration and intensity of the stretches, provided they are pain free.

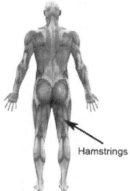

Relevant Anatomy for Hamstring Stretches

Place your foot on a step or chair. Keep your knee and back straight, lean forward at your hips until you feel a stretch in the back of your thigh / knee. Hold for 20 seconds and repeat 4 times at a mild to moderate stretch pain-free.

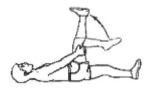

Laying Hamstring Stretch

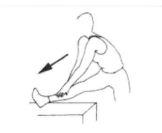

HAMSTRING STRETCH

Foam roller hamstring stretch

Calf Stretch

(Main muscles involved: Gastrocnemius, Soleus, Tibialis Posterior)

The following calf stretches are designed to improve the flexibility of the calf muscles.
To begin with, the calf stretches should be held for 20 seconds and repeated 4 times at a mild to moderate stretch pain free. Generally, you should choose one or two stretches that feel comfortable for you and performed them 3 times daily. As your flexibility improves, the exercises can be progressed by increasing the frequency, duration and intensity of the stretches, provided they are pain free.

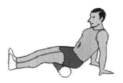

The Calf Muscles

With your hands against the wall, place your leg to be stretched behind you as demonstrated. Keep your heel down, knee straight and feet pointing forwards. Gently lunge forwards until you feel a stretch in the back of your calf / knee. Hold for 20 seconds and repeat 4 times at a mild to moderate stretch pain-free.

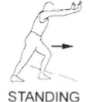

STANDING CALF STRETCH

Calf Stretch

Calf Stretch with Towel

Begin this calf stretch in long sitting with your leg to be stretched in front of you. Your knee and back should be straight and a towel or rigid band placed around your foot as demonstrated. Using your foot, ankle and the towel, bring your toes towards your head until you feel a stretch in the back of your calf, Achilles tendon or leg. Hold for 15 seconds and repeat 4 times at a mild to moderate stretch provided the exercise is pain free.

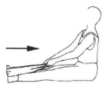

TOWEL STRETCH

Calf Stretch with Towel

Calf Self Massage Exercises

The following calf self-massage exercises are designed to improve the flexibility of the calf muscles and are an excellent addition to the above stretches.

Foam Roller Calf Releases

Place the foam roller under your calves as demonstrated. Using your arms, slowly move your body forward and backwards allowing the foam roller to massage the back of your lower legs. Breathe normally keeping your legs relaxed. Repeat this process for 15 – 90 seconds provided it is comfortable and does not cause pain. This exercise can be progressed by crossing your legs and massaging one calf at a time.

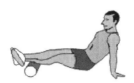

Foam Roller Calf Release

For more info on static stretching and foam rolling, I recommend you to read "Degenerative Disc Disease Pain Relief Plan". It has all the techniques we have covered in this book and more.

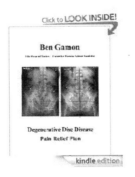

CHAPTER 3: STRENGTHENING EXERCISES

The following leg exercises are designed to improve the strength of the muscles of the legs. Generally, they should only be performed provided they do not cause or increase pain. Begin with the basic leg exercises.

The following basic leg exercises should generally be performed 1 - 3 times per week provided they do not cause or increase pain. Ideally they should not be performed on consecutive days, to allow muscle recovery. As your strength improves, the exercises can be progressed by gradually increasing the repetitions, number of sets or resistance of the leg exercises provided they do not cause or increase pain.

Quadriceps Strengthening Exercises

The following quadriceps strengthening exercises are designed to improve strength of the quadriceps muscle. The quadriceps comprises of four muscle bellies, one of which is the VMO (Vastus Medialis Obliquus). The VMO is very important in quadriceps and knee rehabilitation exercises.

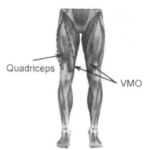

Relevant Anatomy for Quadriceps Strengthening Exercises

Swiss Ball Squats

Begin this leg exercise in standing with your feet shoulder width apart, your feet facing forwards and a Swiss Ball placed between a wall and your back. Slowly perform a squat, keeping your back straight. Your knees should be in line with your middle toes and should not move forward past your toes. Then slowly return to the starting position maintaining good posture throughout the exercise. Perform 1 - 3 sets of 10 repetitions provided the exercise is pain free.

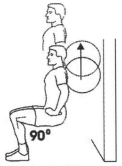
Swiss Ball Squats

Hip Abduction Sidelying
Begin this leg exercise lying on your side in the position demonstrated. Keeping your back and knee straight and foot facing forwards, slowly take your leg upwards tightening the muscles at the side of your thigh / hip (abductors). Hold for 2 seconds and then return to the starting position. Perform 1 – 3 sets of 10 repetitions on each leg provided the exercise is pain free.

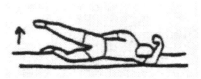
Hip Abduction Side lying (right leg)

Adductor Squeeze
Begin this leg exercise lying on your back in the position demonstrated with a rolled towel or ball between your knees. Slowly squeeze the ball between your knees tightening your inner thigh muscles (adductors). Hold for 5 seconds and then relax. Perform 1 – 3 sets of 10 repetitions provided the exercise is pain free.

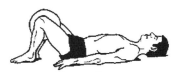
Adductor Squeeze

Resistance Band Knee Extension
Begin this leg exercise in sitting with your knee bent and a resistance band tied around your ankle as shown. Keeping your back straight, slowly straighten your knee, tightening the front of your thigh (quadriceps). Then slowly return to the starting position maintaining good posture throughout the exercise. Perform 1 - 3 sets of 10 repetitions on each leg provided the exercise is pain free.

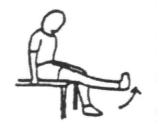

Resistance Band Knee Extension

Resistance Band Knee Flexion

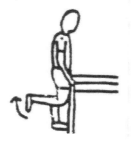

Resistance band hamstring curls / knee flexion

Begin this leg exercise lying on your front with a resistance band tied around your ankle as shown. Slowly bend your knee tightening the muscles at the back of your thigh (hamstrings). Then slowly return to the starting position maintaining good control throughout the exercise. Perform 1 - 3 sets of 10 repetitions on each leg provided the exercise is pain free.

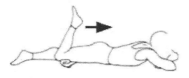

PRONE KNEE FLEXION
Resistance Band Hamstring Curls / knee flexion

CHAPTER 4: HOME TREATMENT

Home treatment helps relieve pain, swelling, and stiffness.

Follow the R.I.C.E method, also explained in "Stress Fracture of The Foot"

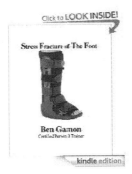

- **REST** and protect an injured or sore area. Stop, change, or take a break from any activity that may be causing your pain or soreness. When resting, place a small pillow under your knee.

- **ICE** will reduce pain and swelling. Apply ice packs or cold packs immediately to prevent or minimize swelling. Apply the ice or cold pack for 10 to 20 minutes, 3 or more times a day. I always recommend the "Peas Cold Therapy" from CVS to my clients.

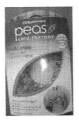

- **COMPRESSION**, or wrapping the injured or sore area with an elastic bandage (such as an Ace wrap), will help decrease swelling. I always recommend my clients to wear an *Ace Knee Brace*. I also have my clients wear a knee brace during their workouts for support.

Don't wrap it too tightly, since this can cause more swelling below the affected area.

- **ELEVATE** the injured or sore area on pillows while applying ice and anytime you are sitting or lying down. Try to keep the area at or above the level of your heart to help minimize swelling.

Medicine you can buy without a prescription:

- Acetaminophen such as Tylenol
- Nonsteroidal anti-inflammatory drugs (NSAID)
    - Ibuprofen, such as Advil or Motrin
    - Naproxen, such Aleve or Naprosyn

- Aspirin (also a nonsteroidal anti-inflammatory drug), such as Bayer or Bufferin
- Glucosamine & Joint Pain

The main function of glucosamine is to help prevent the breakdown of the cartilage between the bones in their joints.

Glucosamine is a naturally occurring substance that is a component of cartilage. Its main function is to help prevent the breakdown of the cartilage between the bones in their joints. Because the knee is a primary site for this breakdown, ensuring the body has a sufficient amount of glucosamine on a regular basis is necessary to both prevent knee injury and promote healthy knee cartilage and joints.

- Dotfit Joint FlexPlus ™

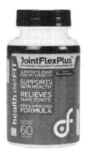

Glucosamine Studies
Many studies have been conducted to evaluate the effect of glucosamine supplement, often along with a similar component called chondroitin sulfate (also a naturally occurring substance), in reducing knee pain and improving the mobility of the knees of people who have osteoarthritis or rheumatoid arthritis. Both glucosamine and chondroitin help keep the cartilage healthy and moist, and when taken in liquid supplement form, can help relieve the pain of osteoarthritis of the knee and may even assist the body in repairing damaged cartilage*.

New & Improved!
The ingredients in Joint Flexibility Plus™ have been shown to support cartilage and joint and skin health. Additionally, the specific ingredients in this formula have been clinically proven to be more than twice as effective as using Glucosamine & Chondroitin Sulfate alone in patients with moderate to severe osteoarthritis. This product has been shown to be well absorbed, tolerated and safe. Proper use of this product may enhance healthy cartilage function.

This product is designed for individuals who want relief of mild joint discomfort with far fewer side effects that occur from chronic non-steroidal anti-inflammatory drug (NSAID) use such as aspirin or ibuprofen.

<u>BioCell Collagen II®</u> *is a multi-patented ingredient that provides a naturally-occurring bioavailable matrix of hydrolyzed collagen type II, hyaluronic acid and chondroitin sulfate, and scientific evidence supports its joint and skin health benefits. BioCell Collagen II® has been clinically shown to help improve joint comfort and mobility*

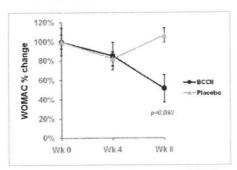

Figure 1: WOMAC scores decreased approx. 50% in the BCCII group but increased 7% in the placebo.

The WOMAC index is used to assess patients with osteoarthritis of the hip or knee using 24 parameters. It can be used to monitor the course of the disease or to determine the effectiveness of anti-rheumatic medications. In this study the WOMAC score measured pain and stiffness in the knee and difficulty in various physical activities. A lower score indicates that the test product has efficacy in improving the symptoms.

Kalman, et al. A randomized double blind clinical trial evaluating the safety and efficacy of hydrolyzed collagen type II in adults with osteoarthritis. LB435, Experimental Biology 2004, Washington, DC.

CHAPTER 5: TRX FOR KNEE REHABILITATION

As most of you know already, the TRX Suspension training is my favorite workout tool. TRX is the acronym for total resistance exercise. All the exercises performed on the TRX keep your core fully engaged. What I love about using TRX with my clients is that it works on their coordination, stability, balance, flexibility, power and strength all at once.

The problem nowadays, and the reason why so many people get injured is because we do not move enough anymore; mostly, we do not really move in three plans of motions.
There are three planes of motions: the sagittal, frontal and transverse plan. Traditional resistance training is not as efficient as the TRX because it only focuses on one plane of motion at a time. The TRX suspension training is not limited to one plan of motion, hence making it more popular.

When performing TRX exercises, neuromuscular responses are generated through gravity and movement. These changes in the body position and joints mechanic result in a resistance, balance and cardio workout. That's why working out with TRX is more efficient than "old traditional workouts". You don't have to do cardio, then resistance training.... You can just spend a little time on the TRX and you will realize how efficient it is, because it combines all types of workouts in one.

If you live in the Los Angeles Area, I strongly encourage you to come try a TRX demo with me. That will change the way you work out forever.

TRX squat

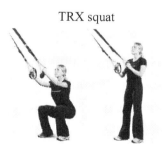

The TRX squat exercise, just as the Swiss ball squat, is a great way to safely strengthen the quadriceps muscle without any impact or added weight on the knees. There are many variations to the TRX squat to develop neuromuscular recruitment and proprioception around the knee.

TRX side lunges

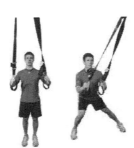

The TRX side lunges are a great way to stretch the back muscles of the extended leg, and strengthen the muscles of the bent leg at the same time.

TRX single leg balance / one leg squat

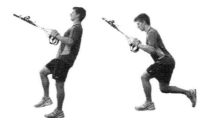

The TRX single leg balance or one leg squat is a progression from the basic TRX squat.

CONCLUSION

I hope you have enjoyed this book and that I have answered some of your questions or concerns regarding knee rehabilitation. The exercises demonstrated in this book are just examples, and you should always seek the advice of a physical therapist or a certified personal trainer that has experience training clients with knee pain.
I invite you to email me at Benjamin.gamon@gmail.com for feedback, questions or comments.

Ben,
Your fitness friend.

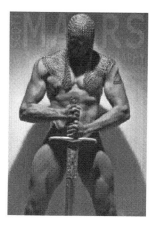

Obviously not a knee rehabilitation exercise; It is just me messing around with my TRX on the streets in San Francisco.

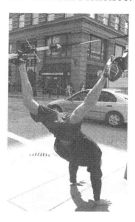

TESTIMONIALS

"I have been training with Ben Gamon for several months. I have worked with countless trainers and coaches over the years and I have to say that Ben is the best I have ever worked with. Ben makes our training sessions fun. We laugh, we joke, we talk about our lives and the ups and downs. One of the main reasons that I have stopped dreading my workouts is because I know I get to spend time with Ben. Not only is he fun to work with, but you can't argue with the results. I have lost 20 lbs in 6 weeks. You have a major asset on your hands with Ben Gamon." "Margot"

"Choosing Ben Gamon as my personal trainer was the best decision I ever made. I was at a point in my work out "career" where I had no motivation left. I just couldn't make it to the gym to save my life (no pun intended). I used every excuse in the book not to go. That is why I chose to hire a personal trainer. Ben really knows his stuff. He safely pushes my body to new levels of strength and endurance. He really tailored my workout to my fitness goals. He's aware of all my "excuses" and pushes me beyond them. I now not only have motivation, I'm addicted." "Joe"

I've been working out with Ben Gamon for 3 months and believe me when I say that he is the best trainer you'll find. He's nothing short of AMAZING. When we first started our sessions I had no idea how much I would grow to respect the effort and time Ben puts into helping me meet my goals. There are days when I'm so tired from work that I don't think I can do it, Ben continues to open my eyes time and again to my potential. He is truly a gifted, inspiring person and an all-around good guy.
"Kalika"

"On a recent visit to San Francisco I decided to train with Ben Gamon. Coming from a background in yoga and pilates I wanted a different approach to fitness. I had high demands I was in town for 4 weeks, I wanted a personal trainer, and I wanted to lose 10 lbs. Without hesitation Ben Gamon took me on and made me work! Each session he pushed me to my edge. He listened to what I wanted and came up with challenging routines to target my goals. Ben exceeded my expectations with his knowledge, patience and ability to always keep our workouts interesting . Combing weight training, boxing, and core work Ben safely pushed me to my physical limits . He used all his knowledge and background in brazilian jujitsu and krav maga to challenge me through each workout, but mostly he broke my excuses and pushed me through my limits! At the end of the four weeks I was amazed at my transformation. My clothing fit better because I have already lost 10lbs.
"Danielle"

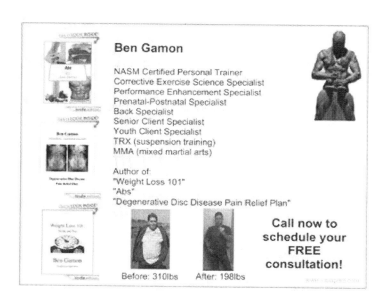

GO FOR IT !!! It is just amazing. This guy is awesome, lots of fun working out with him, his customer service is great and the results on my body are unbelievable. The first month, I gained 7 pounds of muscle, I lost fat and I feel really good now. I have been training with Ben for 9 month, and the only bad thing about that is that I have to buy some new shirts cause I can't fit in the old ones... :-) "John"

"I'd like to shamelessly plug Ben. I've been through a few sessions with Ben and he really helped me bust through a plateau. He is an expert trainer and his knowledge of anatomy, nutrition and all around fitness is impressive. If it's your first time training with a personal trainer in San Francisco, you'll appreciate how Ben finds your physical and mental limits and pushes you well beyond them. You get what you pay for. He also has a positive attitude and is hilarious to talk to. Cheers dude." "Curt"

"I have been training with Ben for over 3 years now. More than my personal trainer, he became one of my best friends." "Marc"

"I've had the privilege of having Ben Gamon as my Personal Trainer for the past 3 years. He really has changed my life. I lost 100lbs of fat, gained muscle mass and greatly improved my physical endurance. I'm in the best shape of my life and I have Ben to thank for that!

My downward spiral, where I began to gain all this weight was a lower back injury. Ben was *able to show me safe exercises that I could do to help strengthen my lower back. Ben's workouts were always hard, but he always watched that I kept the proper form while exercising to keep unnecessary pressure off my lower back.*

Ben has captured his years of training and wisdom in "Weight Loss 101". It's a must read for anyone who is ready to take the challenge of losing weight and improving their lives forever!"

"Mitch"

Mitch before - 310lbs

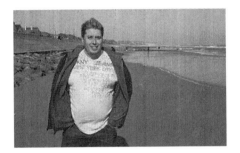

Mitch after - 198lbs

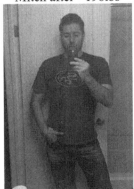

Made in the USA
Lexington, KY
14 March 2012